EVERYTHING ABOUT GALLBLADDER CANCER AND DIETARY CHOICES

Complete Guide To Cholecystitis, Symptoms, Treatment Options, Surgery, Prevention Strategies For Patients And Caregivers

WALTON USELTON

DISCLAIMER

The content in this book is based on the author's expertise and understanding of food and nutrition. The author is not linked or associated with any corporation, business, or person. This book is designed for informative purposes only and should not be interpreted as professional medical advice. Readers should get medical advice before making any changes to their diet or lifestyle. The author takes no responsibility or liability for any repercussions arising from the use of the information included in this book.

ABOUT THIS BOOK

"Gallbladder Cancer And Dietary Choices" is a valuable resource that explores the complex link between food and gallbladder cancer. In its thorough examination, the book guides readers through critical parts of understanding gallbladder cancer, emphasizing the need for early identification and outlining the many treatment options available. Each chapter, from explaining the foundations of the condition to providing dietary suggestions for gallbladder cancer patients, is thoughtfully created to give comprehensive support and insights.

The first part establishes the relevance of dietary choices in controlling gallbladder cancer. It not only explains the risk factors linked with the condition, but it also emphasizes the importance of food in minimizing those risks. Chapter 2 provides readers with vital information on how dietary choices might impact the development and progression of gallbladder cancer. This section not only identifies items that may increase the risk but also provides practical advice on eating a healthy diet to lessen vulnerability.

Chapter 3 guides readers through the nutritional landscape particularly gallbladder cancer, providing vital insights into making dietary adjustments to meet the special demands of individuals undergoing treatment. This chapter serves as a guide for both patients and carers, covering everything from controlling side effects to maintaining proper hydration. In addition, Chapter 4 carefully lists items to avoid, offering insight into dietary behaviors that may worsen the illness. In contrast, Chapter 5 focuses on foods that might serve as the foundation of a gallbladder cancer diet, emphasizing the benefits of fruits, vegetables, healthy grains, and lean protein.

Beyond dietary issues, Chapter 6 looks into complementary and alternative treatments, providing a detailed assessment of their possible advantages and hazards. Furthermore, Chapter 7 emphasizes the necessity of maintaining a holistic lifestyle throughout treatment, highlighting the critical function of exercise, stress management, and social support networks. Chapter 8 dives into coping methods for nutritional problems, offering practical ways for both patients and carers to deal with changes in appetite and taste.

Transitioning to life after cancer treatment, Chapter 9 discusses survivability, lobbying for frequent follow-up visits, and long-term nutritional attention. Finally, Chapter 10 lifts the discussion by calling for awareness and prevention, emphasizing the need for community responsibility in promoting cancer prevention measures and assisting people in taking control of their health.

"Gallbladder Cancer And Dietary Choices" is more than just a collection of facts; it is a source of hope, empowerment, and education for those dealing with gallbladder cancer. With its expertly crafted information and steadfast devotion to holistic well-being, this book is an essential resource for patients, carers, and healthcare professionals alike.

INTRODUCTION

Understanding Gallbladder Cancer

Gallbladder cancer, although relatively uncommon, maybe a dangerous illness that needs careful monitoring and treatment. The gallbladder is a tiny organ under the liver that stores bile, which aids with digestion. Cancer in gallbladder tissues may cause a variety of consequences and health problems.

Overview Of Gallbladder Cancer

Gallbladder cancer usually begins in the gallbladder's innermost layer and may spread to other areas of the organ or adjacent lymph nodes. The signs of gallbladder cancer may be subtle in the early stages, making diagnosis difficult. However, when the disease develops, patients may feel stomach discomfort, jaundice, nausea, and weight loss.

Risk Factors Associated With The Disease

Several factors may raise the chance of acquiring gallbladder cancer. These include age, which increases the danger as people become older. Other risk factors include feminine gender, a history of gallstones or gallbladder polyps, obesity, certain genetic disorders, and exposure to certain chemicals or poisons.

The Importance Of Early Detection

Early identification of gallbladder cancer is critical for enhancing treatment results and increasing the likelihood of full recovery. Unfortunately, since symptoms often develop after the disease has progressed, many patients are not recognized until later stages. Individuals who are at risk should get frequent tests and be aware of any possible signs.

Diet In Managing Gallbladder Cancer

Diet is an important part of controlling gallbladder cancer and may help improve overall health and quality of life for those who have the illness. A balanced diet may offer critical nutrients, boost the immune system, and assist manage treatment-related symptoms and adverse effects.

The Purpose Of The Book

The goal of this book is to give thorough information and practical advice on dietary options for those who have gallbladder cancer. Understanding the importance of food in cancer management allows readers to make educated nutrition and lifestyle choices that will support their health and well-being throughout their cancer journey. This book attempts to empower readers to take control of their food and optimize their nutrition to improve their overall quality of life while living with gallbladder cancer.

CHAPTER ONE

Basics Of Gallbladder Cancer

What Is Gallbladder Cancer?

Gallbladder cancer begins in the tissues of the gallbladder, a tiny organ found under the liver. It is a very uncommon kind of cancer, but it may be aggressive and difficult to treat, especially because it is often identified at an advanced stage. The gallbladder stores bile generated by the liver for digestion. Cancer may grow in any area of the gallbladder, although it most often begins in the organ's inner lining.

Types And Stages Of Gallbladder Cancer

Gallbladder cancer is classified into numerous forms, the most frequent of which is adenocarcinoma. Squamous cell carcinoma, adenosquamous carcinoma, and small cell carcinoma are among the less prevalent varieties. These kinds change depending on the exact cells in which the cancer begins.

Gallbladder cancer is further classified into phases depending on tumor size, extent of dissemination, and metastasis to other areas of the body. Staging assists in determining the optimal treatment option and prognosis for the patient. Early-stage tumors are limited to the gallbladder's inner layers, whereas advanced-stage malignancies have progressed outside the organ to adjacent lymph nodes or other organs.

Symptoms And Diagnoses

Gallbladder cancer symptoms are generally vague and nonspecific, mirroring those of other digestive diseases. These symptoms might include stomach discomfort, bloating, nausea, vomiting, jaundice (yellowing of the skin and eyes), and unexplained weight loss.

Because these symptoms may be caused by a variety of illnesses, gallbladder cancer is often discovered after it has progressed to an advanced stage.

Gallbladder cancer is often diagnosed using a mix of imaging tests, including ultrasound, CT scans, and MRI scans, to see the gallbladder and surrounding tissues. Blood tests may also be performed to look for signs that suggest malignancy. In certain situations, a biopsy may be required to confirm the diagnosis by analyzing a sample of tissue under a microscope.

Importance Of Early Detection

Early identification of gallbladder cancer is critical for enhancing treatment results and survival rates. Unfortunately, since symptoms are typically ambiguous and the illness is very uncommon, gallbladder cancer is frequently detected at an advanced stage, with few treatment choices. That is why those who are suffering symptoms like stomach discomfort, jaundice, or unexplained weight loss should seek medical assistance right once.

Regular check-ups with a healthcare professional may also help with early diagnosis, particularly for those who are at a greater risk owing to factors including a history of gallstones, chronic gallbladder inflammation, or certain genetic diseases. By finding gallbladder cancer early, clinicians may investigate a broader variety of treatment options, such as surgery, chemotherapy, and radiation therapy, to improve patient outcomes.

Treatment Alternatives Are Available

The treatment technique for gallbladder cancer is determined by various aspects, including the stage of the illness, the patient's general health, and their preferences. Surgery is the main therapy for early-stage gallbladder cancer, with choices ranging from gallbladder removal (cholecystectomy) to more elaborate operations that may include the removal of adjacent lymph nodes, sections of the liver, or bile ducts.

When surgery alone is ineffective, further therapies such as chemotherapy or radiation therapy may be prescribed to reduce tumors, kill residual cancer cells, or ease symptoms. These therapies may be administered before or after surgery to help control the tumor and minimize the chance of recurrence.

Advanced-stage gallbladder cancer that has spread to other regions of the body is treated with palliative care to manage symptoms and improve quality of life. This might include pain management, nutritional assistance, and other treatments targeted at alleviating suffering and improving well-being.

Individuals with gallbladder cancer may also participate in clinical trials, which provide access to novel medicines and therapies that are still in the experimental stage. Participating in clinical trials may give patients access to cutting-edge care while also helping to increase medical understanding and treatment choices for gallbladder cancer.

Overall, gallbladder cancer therapy is difficult and often requires a collaborative effort among a variety of healthcare providers, including surgeons, medical oncologists, radiation oncologists, and supportive care specialists. Healthcare practitioners may assist people with gallbladder cancer to achieve the best possible results and retain the greatest quality of life by collaborating to personalize treatment strategies to each patient's specific requirements and circumstances.

CHAPTER TWO

The Relationship Between Diet And Gallbladder Cancer

Exploring The Relationship Between Diet And Cancer

Understanding the link between nutrition and gallbladder cancer is critical for both prevention and treatment. While genetics and environmental variables are important, a new study shows that dietary choices can influence gallbladder health. Individuals who investigate this connection may make more educated choices to lower their risk or successfully manage the disease.

According to studies, certain eating habits may lead to the development of gallbladder cancer. For example, diets heavy in saturated fats, refined carbohydrates, and processed foods have been related to an increased risk. These foods may cause obesity, diabetes, and other metabolic diseases, all of which are risk factors for gallbladder cancer. Furthermore, a low-fiber diet may decrease gallbladder function and raise the risk of cancer.

Adopting a diet high in fruits, vegetables, whole grains, and lean meats, on the other hand, may help minimize your risk of gallbladder cancer. These foods provide critical nutrients, antioxidants, and fiber, which promote general health and may help prevent cancer formation. Understanding these dietary trends allows people to make proactive decisions that enhance gallbladder health.

Effect Of Diet On Gallbladder Health

Diet has an influence on gallbladder health that is not limited to cancer risk. Certain foods may affect gallbladder function and the production of gallstones, a frequent precursor to gallbladder cancer. For example, high-cholesterol and saturated fat diets may contribute to gallstone development by raising cholesterol levels in bile, causing cholesterol particles to crystallize.

Furthermore, rapid weight loss or frequent fasting might increase the risk of gallstone development since the gallbladder may not empty effectively without regular food intake. A balanced diet, on the other hand, that contains healthy fats, moderate protein, and enough water, may help the gallbladder operate properly and lower the chance of gallstone formation.

Understanding how various dietary components impact gallbladder health enables people to make more educated decisions that assist preventative and treatment efforts. Individuals may take proactive actions to minimize their chance of getting gallbladder cancer by eating foods that support gallbladder health while avoiding those that may damage it.

Foods That Might Increase The Risk Of Gallbladder Cancer

Certain foods and dietary habits have been linked to an increased risk of gallbladder cancer. This includes:

1. **High-Fat Diets:** Consuming saturated and trans fats, such as fried meals, fatty cuts of meat, and processed snacks, may increase the risk of gallbladder cancer. These fats may cause obesity and metabolic problems, both of which are risk factors for cancer development.

2. Foods heavy in refined sugars and carbs, such as sugary beverages, white bread, and pastries, may raise blood sugar levels and cause inflammation, thus raising the risk of gallbladder cancer over time.

3. **Processed Meats:** Eating processed meats such as bacon, sausage, and deli meats has been related to an increased risk of many malignancies, including

gallbladder cancer. These meats often include chemicals and preservatives, which may lead to cancer development.

4. Low-Fiber Diets: Diets deficient in fiber from fruits, vegetables, and whole grains may impair gallbladder function and increase the risk of gallstone development, a precursor to gallbladder cancer.

Foods That May Reduce The Risk Of Gallbladder Cancer

In contrast, some foods and dietary habits may help reduce the incidence of gallbladder cancer. This includes:

1. Fruits and vegetables are high in antioxidants, vitamins, and fiber, which help to prevent cancer. Consuming a range of colorful fruits and vegetables may give critical nutrients for general health and may lower the chance of gallbladder cancer.

2. Whole grains, such as brown rice, quinoa, and whole wheat, include fiber and other nutrients that improve digestive health and may help reduce gallstone development. Whole grains may increase satiety and minimize the intake of refined carbs.

3. **Lean Proteins:** Choosing lean protein sources like chicken, fish, beans, and lentils over red and processed meats will help lower your risk of gallbladder cancer. These protein alternatives include less saturated fat and offer critical nutrients without the negative consequences associated with processed meats.

4. **Healthy Fats:** Consuming healthy fats from sources such as olive oil, avocado, nuts, and seeds helps improve gallbladder health and decrease inflammation in the body. These fats provide important fatty acids that are required for cellular function and may help reduce the risk of gallbladder cancer when ingested in moderation.

Importance Of Keeping A Healthy Diet

Maintaining a balanced diet is critical for general health, including gallbladder function. Individuals may lower their chance of acquiring gallbladder cancer and other associated disorders by adopting informed dietary choices. Incorporating a range of nutrient-dense foods, avoiding excessive use of hazardous substances, and eating a well-balanced diet may all help to support normal gallbladder function and enhance overall health. Prioritizing a balanced diet, as well as frequent physical exercise and other lifestyle changes may help prevent cancer and improve overall health.

Chapter THREE

Nutritional Guidelines For Gallbladder Cancer Patients

Understanding Nutritional Needs For Cancer Treatment

Nutrition is essential for controlling gallbladder cancer, particularly during therapy. Understanding your body's dietary requirements may help relieve symptoms, strengthen your immune system, and enhance your general quality of life during this difficult time.

When receiving cancer therapy, your body may need additional nutrients to aid in healing, combat infection, and maintain energy levels. However, cancer and its therapies may have an impact on your appetite, digestion, and capacity to absorb nutrients, so it's critical to consume nutrient-dense, easily digestible meals.

Managing Side Effects Of Treatment Through Diet

Chemotherapy, radiation treatment, and surgery may all have adverse impacts on your capacity to consume and digest food. Common side effects include nausea, vomiting, diarrhea, constipation, mouth sores, and taste alterations, which may make it difficult to stick to a balanced eating plan.

To treat these side effects, try dietary changes that target your symptoms. If you're feeling nauseous, basic meals like crackers, rice, and bananas may be easier to stomach. Drinking ginger tea and nibbling on ginger candies might also help with nausea.

Soft, mild meals such as yogurt, mashed potatoes, and scrambled eggs may help with mouth sores. Avoiding hot, acidic, or rough-textured meals might help avoid additional aggravation.

Recommended Dietary Modifications For Gallbladder Cancer Patients

Gallbladder cancer and its therapies may alter how your body absorbs certain nutrients, so it is important to adopt dietary changes that promote your health and well-being. Here are some broad recommendations:

1. Limiting Fat consumption: Because the gallbladder helps digest fats, you may need to limit your fat consumption if you've had surgery to remove it or if it's not working correctly. Choose lean proteins such as chicken, fish, and tofu, and moderately consume healthy fats such as avocados, nuts, and seeds.

2. Increasing Fibre: Fiber-rich meals may help reduce constipation, which is a typical side effect of cancer

therapy and several pain drugs. Include fruits, vegetables, whole grains, and legumes in your diet to guarantee appropriate fiber consumption.

3. **Sugar Intake**: Some cancer therapies, notably steroids, might raise blood sugar levels. Limiting your consumption of sugary meals and drinks will help you maintain stable blood sugar levels and avoid energy dumps.

4. Protein is required for tissue regeneration and immunological function, both of which are critical during cancer therapy. Poultry, fish, eggs, dairy, beans, and lentils are good sources of lean protein.

Importance Of Hydration And Fluid Intake

Staying hydrated is essential for dealing with the adverse effects of cancer therapy and maintaining general health.

Chemotherapy and radiation treatment might raise the risk of dehydration owing to nausea, vomiting, diarrhea, and reduced appetite.

To keep hydrated, consume lots of fluids throughout the day, such as water, herbal teas, broth-based soups, and diluted fruit juices. Avoid caffeinated and alcoholic drinks, which may lead to dehydration.

If you're having difficulties drinking enough fluids, try sipping tiny quantities regularly, using a straw, or flavoring your water with lemon or cucumber slices to help it taste better.

Tips On Meal Planning And Preparation

Meal planning and preparation may assist in guaranteeing that you obtain enough nutrition while dealing with the demands of cancer treatment. Here are some suggestions to ease the process:

1. **Plan:** Set aside some time each week to plan your meals and snacks. Consider making big amounts of meals that can be portioned and refrigerated for convenient reheating.

2. **Choose** nutrient-dense meals to increase your consumption of vitamins, minerals, and antioxidants. Include a wide range of fruits, vegetables, whole grains, lean meats, and healthy fats in your meals.

3. **Make Simple Swaps:** If specific meals are causing pain or digestive concerns, consider replacing them with more tolerable alternatives. For example, if dairy products affect you, consider lactose-free alternatives such as almond milk or coconut yogurt.

4. **Listen to Your Body:** Consider how various meals make you feel and change your diet appropriately. If you're suffering particular symptoms, such as nausea or diarrhea, consider changing your diet to see if it relieves your discomfort.

Understanding your nutritional needs, managing treatment side effects through diet, making recommended dietary changes, prioritizing hydration, and implementing practical meal planning and preparation tips will help you maintain your health and well-being throughout your gallbladder cancer journey.

CHAPTER FOUR

Foods To Avoid For Gallbladder Cancer Patients

High-Fat Foods And Their Effect On Gallbladder Health

When dealing with gallbladder cancer, it is critical to monitor the kinds of fats you ingest. High-fat diets may worsen gallbladder problems and raise the risk of complications. Saturated and trans fats, which are often found in fried meals, processed snacks, and fatty meats, should be reduced or avoided completely. These lipids may form gallstones and cause inflammation in the gallbladder, thereby aggravating cancer patients' conditions.

Choose healthy fats, such as those found in avocados, nuts, seeds, and fatty seafood like salmon, to supply necessary nutrients without placing excessive pressure on your gallbladder. These fats include omega-3 fatty acids, which have anti-inflammatory qualities and may help manage gallbladder cancer symptoms.

Processed Foods And Their Relationship With Cancer Risk

Processed foods are often loaded with chemicals, preservatives, and bad fats, making them harmful to general health, particularly for those who have gallbladder cancer. These foods have been related to a higher risk of several malignancies, including gallbladder cancer. Processed foods have high quantities of salt, sugar, and harmful fats, which may cause inflammation, weight gain, and poor digestion, all of which can aggravate symptoms and impair the prognosis for cancer patients.

Instead of processed meals, aim to include complete, natural foods in your diet. Fresh fruits and vegetables, whole grains, lean meats, and healthy fats should be the foundations of your diet. Not only will this improve your general health and well-being, but it may also give critical minerals and antioxidants that may assist with cancer therapy and recovery.

Limit Or Avoid Foods That Are High In Sugar And Calories

Excess sugar intake has been related to a wide range of health problems, including obesity, diabetes, and cancer. Individuals with gallbladder cancer should restrict or avoid high-calorie and sugary meals to assist in controlling symptoms and promote overall health. Sugary sweets such as cakes, cookies, candies, and sugary beverages are high in empty calories and may lead to weight gain, insulin resistance, and inflammation, all of which can have a detrimental influence on cancer treatment results.

Instead of going for sugary foods, choose naturally sweet options such as fresh fruit, unsweetened yogurt, or dark chocolate in moderation. Furthermore, keep track of your total calorie consumption and strive to maintain a healthy weight via balanced meals and frequent physical exercise. This may assist increase energy levels, immunological function, and general quality of life while undergoing cancer therapy.

Red Meat's Potential Role In Cancer Development

While red meat may provide protein and vital minerals, excessive intake has been associated with an increased risk of many malignancies, including gallbladder cancer. Red meat is heavy in saturated fat and cholesterol, which may cause inflammation and oxidative stress in the body, thus increasing cancer development and progression.

Individuals with gallbladder cancer should reduce their intake of red meat and instead consume leaner protein sources such as chicken, fish, beans, and lentils. These alternatives provide comparable nutritional advantages without the additional dangers linked with red meat. Incorporating more plant-based meals into your diet may also give health advantages such as lower inflammation, better digestion, and increased immunological function.

Alcohol Use And Its Effects On Gallbladder Cancer

Alcohol intake may be harmful to gallbladder health and may increase symptoms for those with gallbladder cancer. Alcohol is known to irritate the digestive tract's lining, especially the gallbladder, causing inflammation and increasing the risk of issues including gallstones and bile duct blockage. Furthermore, excessive alcohol intake has been related to an increased risk of many malignancies, particularly gut cancers.

If you have gallbladder cancer, you should restrict or eliminate alcohol to reduce further pressure on your digestive system and improve overall health. Instead of alcoholic drinks, choose hydrating options such as water, herbal teas, or freshly squeezed juice. These products not only help you stay hydrated, but they also include critical minerals and antioxidants that may improve your body's natural healing processes. Making attentive eating choices and prioritizing your health may help you manage symptoms and improve results throughout cancer treatment.

CHAPTER FIVE

Foods For A Gallbladder Cancer Diet

Fruits And Vegetables Have An Important Role In Cancer Prevention

Fruits and vegetables are crucial components of a gallbladder cancer diet because they provide several health advantages, including cancer prevention. These natural foods are high in vitamins, minerals, antioxidants, and dietary fiber, all of which help to maintain general health and strengthen the body's defenses against malignant cells.

Incorporating a variety of colorful fruits and vegetables into your daily diet may offer a broad range of nutrients that strengthen your immune system and lower your chance of developing cancer.

Berries, such as strawberries, blueberries, and raspberries, are high in antioxidants such as anthocyanins and flavonoids, which have been linked to a decreased risk of cancer by neutralizing damaging free radicals in the body.

Cruciferous plants such as broccoli, kale, and cauliflower are also very useful to gallbladder cancer patients because of their high concentration of sulfur-containing chemicals known as glucosinolates. These chemicals have been demonstrated to have anti-cancer characteristics because they limit the development of cancer cells and promote their removal from the body.

Furthermore, fruits and vegetables are low in calories and high in dietary fiber, which may help with weight loss and improve good digestion—an important element of treating gallbladder cancer symptoms and side effects.

Whole Grains And Their Function In A Healthy Diet

Whole grains are an important part of a gallbladder cancer diet since they provide several health advantages in addition to cancer prevention. Unlike processed grains such as white rice and white bread, whole grains maintain their bran and germ layers, which are high in fiber, vitamins, minerals, and antioxidants.

Whole grains, such as brown rice, quinoa, oats, and whole wheat bread, may help manage blood sugar levels, decrease inflammation, and promote heart health—all of which are crucial for general well-being, particularly for cancer patients.

Whole grains include fiber, which improves digestion and increases satiety, keeping you satisfied for longer periods and thus reducing overeating or unhealthy snacking.

Furthermore, the complex carbohydrates included in whole grains give a consistent supply of energy, which is excellent for gallbladder cancer patients who are fatigued or weak as a result of their disease or therapy.

Lean Protein Sources For Gallbladder Cancer Patients

Protein is a vital ingredient for the body's development, repair, and immunological function, therefore it's an important part of a gallbladder cancer diet. However, it is important to choose lean protein sources that supply the required nutrients without excessive saturated fat or cholesterol, which might aggravate some health issues or raise cancer risk.

Choose lean protein sources such as skinless chicken, fish, tofu, lentils, and low-fat dairy products to satisfy your protein requirements while reducing bad fats.

Fish, in particular, is high in omega-3 fatty acids, which have been linked to decreased inflammation and better overall health outcomes, including a reduced chance of cancer development.

Including a range of lean protein sources in your diet will also assist ensure that you're receiving all of the key amino acids your body needs for maximum performance since various protein sources have varied amino acid profiles.

Plant-Based Alternatives To Animal Products

There are many nutritional options available for gallbladder cancer patients who want to minimize their intake of animal products or switch to a more plant-based diet. Plant-based protein sources such as beans, lentils, chickpeas, tofu, tempeh, and seitan may supply enough protein while avoiding the saturated fat and cholesterol present in many animal products.

In addition, plant-based foods such as nuts, seeds, and nut butter include healthy fats, protein, and a range of critical elements that promote general health and well-being. Incorporating these plant-based alternatives into your meals will help vary your diet, satisfy nutritional demands, and reduce your dependency on animal products.

Furthermore, plant-based diets have been linked to a variety of health advantages, including a decreased risk of chronic illnesses such as cancer, heart disease, and diabetes. You may construct a nutritious diet by concentrating on whole, plant-based meals while limiting processed foods and added sugars.

Herbs And Spices With Possible Anti-Cancer Properties

In addition to fruits, vegetables, nutritious grains, and lean meats, herbs and spices with anti-cancer qualities may help support a gallbladder cancer diet.

Many herbs and spices include bioactive chemicals that have antioxidant, anti-inflammatory, and anti-cancer properties, making them effective complements to a cancer-fighting diet.

Turmeric, for example, includes curcumin, a substance with strong anti-inflammatory and antioxidant effects that has been investigated for its possible involvement in cancer prevention and therapy. Similarly, ginger has been proven to have anti-cancer characteristics, such as suppressing cancer cell development and triggering apoptosis (programmed cell death).

Other herbs and spices, such as garlic, cinnamon, oregano, and basil, have chemicals that, when combined with a balanced diet, may help lower the risk of cancer and improve general health. Experimenting with various herbs and spices in your cooking may not only improve the flavor of your food, but it also has possible health advantages that may help you fight gallbladder cancer.

CHAPTER SIX

Supplements And Alternative Therapies

An Overview Of Supplements Often Utilized By Cancer Patients

Supplements have received a lot of attention as adjuncts to established cancer therapies, particularly in situations like gallbladder cancer, where dietary choices are critical. Vitamins, minerals, herbs, and other natural goods are among the most common supplements. Vitamin D, for example, is often advised for its possible involvement in immune function and bone health. Antioxidants such as vitamins C and E are also popular because of their claimed capacity to combat oxidative stress, which has been related to cancer formation. Minerals like selenium and zinc are thought to improve immune function and decrease inflammation, whilst herbs like turmeric and green tea extract are recognized for their anti-inflammatory and antioxidant qualities.

However, it is important to understand that supplements are not without danger. Certain supplements, whether taken in large quantities or conjunction with other drugs, might interfere with cancer therapies or worsen adverse effects. For example, excessive vitamin E dosages may raise the risk of bleeding, which might be troublesome during surgery or chemotherapy. Similarly, certain plants may interact with chemotherapy medications, lowering their efficacy or increasing their toxicity. Thus, although supplements may have potential advantages, they should be used carefully and under the supervision of a healthcare practitioner.

Potential Advantages And Hazards Of Using Supplements

The use of supplements in cancer treatment is a hotly debated issue, owing to the possible advantages and hazards. On the one hand, supplements may help correct nutritional deficiencies, reduce treatment side effects, and promote general health and well-being throughout cancer treatment. For example, omega-3 fatty acids contained in fish oil supplements may assist cancer patients decrease inflammation and enhance their appetite. Similarly, probiotics may help manage gastrointestinal adverse effects associated with chemotherapy or radiation treatment.

However, supplement usage may be dangerous, especially when taken in large dosages or without medical supervision. Some supplements may interfere with cancer therapies, lowering their efficacy or exacerbating the negative effects. Antioxidants, such as vitamins C and E, may interfere with the oxidative stress processes used by certain chemotherapy treatments to destroy cancer cells. Furthermore, many vitamins and minerals, when consumed in excess, may be poisonous to the body and cause damage rather than good. For example, large dosages of vitamin A may induce liver damage, but high selenium consumption can produce selenosis, a disorder characterized by hair loss, exhaustion, and neurological difficulties.

Alternative Therapies: Their Role In Cancer Treatment

Alternative therapies refer to a broad variety of practices and interventions performed in addition to or instead of traditional cancer treatments. Acupuncture, massage treatment, meditation, yoga, and nutritional supplements are some of the possible remedies. Some alternative medicines try to manage symptoms and improve quality of life, while others promise to cure cancer.

However, data on the effectiveness of alternative cancer treatments is often weak and contentious.

Acupuncture is a popular alternative treatment in recent years. Some studies show that acupuncture may assist with cancer-related pain, nausea, and exhaustion, but additional study is required to validate these results. Similarly, massage therapy has been demonstrated to lower anxiety and increase mood in cancer patients, offering important emotional support throughout treatment. Mind-body techniques such as meditation and yoga are also becoming recognized for their potential advantages in stress reduction, sleep improvement, and general well-being.

Importance Of Consulting Healthcare Professionals Before Using Supplements

Before introducing supplements or alternative treatments into their cancer treatment plan, patients should always check with their healthcare provider.

Oncologists, nutritionists, and integrative medicine experts may provide advice and assistance depending on a patient's medical history, treatment plan, and dietary requirements. They may assist patients in navigating the complicated terrain of supplements, ensuring that they make educated, safe, and suitable selections for their unique condition.

Consulting with healthcare specialists is especially crucial since supplements and alternative therapies might interact with cancer treatments, possibly reducing their effectiveness or safety. Certain herbs, for example, may interact with chemotherapy medications, lowering their efficacy or raising their toxicity. Similarly, large amounts of vitamins or minerals may induce severe responses or unanticipated side effects, particularly in people with underlying health issues or weakened immune systems. Patients who engage closely with their healthcare team may reduce risks and maximize the potential advantages of supplements and alternative treatments in cancer treatment.

Integrative Approaches To Cancer Care

Integrative cancer care combines traditional medical treatments with complementary therapies to address the physical, emotional, and spiritual dimensions of recovery. This holistic approach incorporates evidence-based supplementary therapies such as dietary counseling, exercise programs, stress management strategies, and mind-body practices to assist the complete person rather than merely treat the condition.

Nutrition counseling is an important part of integrative cancer care, helping patients optimize their nutrition to improve treatment results and general health. Dietitians may provide personalized nutrition recommendations based on the patient's requirements, including nutritional status, treatment side effects, and dietary preferences. Exercise programs may also aid with physical function, tiredness reduction, and quality of life before and after cancer treatment.

Stress management strategies, such as mindfulness-based stress reduction and relaxation therapy, may also help to alleviate the emotional and psychological effects of cancer. These methods aid patients in dealing with anxiety, sadness, and other mental health issues that often accompany cancer diagnosis and treatment. By incorporating these alternative therapies into traditional cancer care, patients may benefit from a more thorough and holistic approach to healing that meets their specific needs and promotes general well-being during cancer treatment.

CHAPTER SEVEN

Maintaining A Healthy Lifestyle Throughout Treatment

The Value Of Regular Exercise For Cancer Patients

Regular exercise is essential for cancer patients, particularly those with gallbladder cancer. While exercising during treatment may seem paradoxical, it may have a variety of advantages. First and foremost, exercise helps to preserve strength and endurance, which might be depleted after cancer therapy. It may also boost mood, decrease tiredness, and increase general quality of life.

The kind and intensity of exercise for gallbladder cancer patients might vary based on their specific circumstances and treatment regimens. Consult with healthcare providers to create a personalized workout regimen that takes into consideration your current fitness level, medication side effects, and any physical constraints.

Walking, swimming, yoga, and light stretching routines are all appropriate workouts for persons with gallbladder cancer. These exercises may be tailored to suit individual talents and tastes. Start softly and progressively raise the intensity as acceptable. Even little periods of exercise may be helpful, so finding ways to move throughout the day is essential.

Tips To Manage Stress And Anxiety During Treatment

Managing stress and anxiety is critical for gallbladder cancer patients receiving therapy. Stress influences not just emotional well-being, but also physical health and treatment results. Fortunately, there are various ways to reduce stress and promote relaxation.

Deep breathing exercises are an efficient strategy for calming the mind and reducing stress in the body. Mindfulness and meditation may also help patients create a feeling of serenity and presence in the face of treatment hurdles. Furthermore, indulging in fun activities such as hobbies, spending time with loved ones, or listening to music may bring much-needed diversion and emotional comfort.

Patients should talk freely with their healthcare team about any stress or worry they are experiencing. Counseling, support groups, and relaxation treatments may be provided to assist patients in dealing with emotional discomfort while undergoing treatment.

Quality Sleep And Its Effect On Cancer Recovery

Quality sleep is crucial in cancer rehabilitation, particularly for gallbladder cancer patients. Adequate rest is required for the body to repair and renew cells, and this is especially critical during therapy when the body is stressed. However, cancer and its treatment may often affect sleep patterns, resulting in symptoms such as insomnia or exhaustion.

Setting up a regular nighttime routine will help you sleep better. This might involve reading, having a warm bath, or practicing relaxation methods before bedtime. Creating a pleasant sleep environment devoid of distractions, such as electronic gadgets or excessive noise, may also help with sleep quality.

Patients with gallbladder cancer who are having sleep difficulties should consult with their healthcare practitioners. They may provide recommendations for addressing symptoms like pain or discomfort that might disrupt sleep, as well as drugs or behavioral therapy to enhance sleep quality.

Social Networks For Cancer Patients

Social support is crucial to gallbladder cancer patients as they navigate the hurdles of diagnosis and therapy. A robust support network of family, friends, and healthcare professionals may provide emotional comfort, practical aid, and vital information throughout the cancer treatment process.

Maintaining open communication with loved ones about their thoughts, worries, and wants is critical for creating a supportive atmosphere. This may include expressing thanks for the support received and being open about the effect of cancer on everyday life. Seeking out support groups or online communities may also link patients with people who understand their situations and give encouragement and solidarity.

Healthcare practitioners may also give valuable support and information to gallbladder cancer patients and their families. They may provide information about treatment alternatives, symptom management measures, and further support services.

Mind-Body Practices For Holistic Wellness

Integrating mind-body techniques into everyday living may help gallbladder cancer sufferers achieve overall well-being. These practices acknowledge the interdependence of the mind, body, and spirit, and they seek to promote balance and harmony in all areas of life.

Yoga is a popular mind-body exercise that incorporates physical postures, breathwork, and meditation to help people relax and reduce stress. Yoga has been found in studies to increase mood, decrease anxiety, and improve overall quality of life in cancer patients.

Tai chi, a gentle martial art that emphasizes slow, flowing motions and deep breathing, is also a helpful exercise. Tai chi has been demonstrated to increase balance, strength, and flexibility, making it ideal for cancer patients who may be physically limited or fatigued.

Simple daily activities such as spending time in nature, practicing gratitude, and participating in creative expression, in addition to formal mind-body practices, may all contribute to overall well-being. The aim is to choose practices that correspond to individual tastes and requirements and apply them to everyday life to promote general health and healing.

CHAPTER EIGHT

Coping With Dietary Challenges

Managing Hunger And Taste Changes During Therapy

Managing changes in appetite and taste after gallbladder cancer therapy may be difficult, but there are techniques to assist. Many patients' sense of taste changes, ranging from metallic to total loss of flavor. Furthermore, appetite changes are normal, with some people having a reduced appetite and others having an increased hunger.

To cope with these changes, it's necessary to try new meals and flavors to see what's manageable and appealing. Some people find that cold or room-temperature meals are easier to handle than hot ones, while others prefer bland foods that cause less nausea or discomfort.

For people who are experiencing taste changes, adding herbs and spices to foods might help accentuate the flavors.

Maintaining a sufficient diet throughout treatment is critical to overall health and well-being. Even if your appetite is low, it is important to eat nutrient-dense meals to supply your body with the energy and resources it needs to recover and fight cancer. Small, frequent meals or snacks may be easier to manage than big meals, and nutritional supplements may assist address dietary gaps.

Strategies For Treating Nausea And Digestive Problems

Nausea and digestive problems are frequent adverse effects of gallbladder cancer and therapy. To reduce these symptoms, identify and eliminate causes wherever feasible.

Certain foods or scents may cause nausea in certain people, so maintaining a food diary might help identify possible triggers.

Eating small, frequent meals throughout the day may also help to reduce nausea and stomach pain. Rice, bananas, and bread are all easy to digest. Ginger, whether ingested as tea, capsules or as a snack, has anti-nausea qualities that may help some people.

Staying hydrated is essential, but it's better to consume fluids steadily throughout the day rather than in huge quantities at once, which may exacerbate nausea. Avoiding fatty, oily, or spicy meals may also aid with digestive troubles, since they are more difficult for the body to process, particularly if the gallbladder is impaired.

Meal Planning Tips For Carers And Family Members

Carers and family members play an important role in assisting patients undergoing gallbladder cancer treatment, including food planning and preparation. When arranging meals, it is important to consider the patient's dietary preferences and constraints. This might include cooking smaller servings or changing recipes to meet variations in appetite and taste.

Consuming a diverse range of nutrient-dense meals is critical for sustaining general health and boosting the immune system. Aim to eat a variety of lean proteins, fruits, vegetables, whole grains, and healthy fats in each meal. When feasible, include the person in meal preparation to ensure that their preferences and requirements are considered.

Meal planning may be eased by bulk preparing and storing meals for later use. This not only saves time but also guarantees that nutritional meals are always accessible, even on days when energy levels are low or symptoms are very difficult. Furthermore, having a supply of easy-to-prepare snacks and meals on hand may help reduce stress and ensure that the client receives the nutrition they need.

Seeking Help From Healthcare Experts And Dietitians

Navigating nutritional problems during gallbladder cancer treatment may be intimidating, but healthcare experts and nutritionists are there to help. These professionals may provide tailored advice and suggestions based on specific requirements and preferences.

Using medication and other measures, healthcare practitioners may assist control symptoms such as nausea, vomiting, and digestive difficulties.

They may also monitor nutritional status and give suggestions for dietary changes or supplementation as necessary.

Nutritionists may provide personalized meal plans and nutritional guidance to ensure that patients get enough nourishment to maintain their overall health and well-being throughout treatment. They may also address particular problems, such as weight loss or malnutrition, and provide techniques for improving nutritional intake.

The Significance Of Keeping A Good Attitude Regarding Food And Nutrition

Maintaining a good attitude towards food and nutrition is critical for general health while undergoing gallbladder cancer therapy. While dietary issues may emerge, approaching food with a positive and grateful attitude may help relieve stress and improve the eating experience.

Focusing on the nutritious elements of food, such as its capacity to offer energy and promote healing, may help transform the mindset from annoyance to thankfulness. Experimenting with different flavors and recipes, even in tiny quantities, may bring excitement to meals and improve the eating experience.

Mindful eating habits, such as savoring each meal and paying attention to hunger and fullness signals, may help you develop a healthy connection with food. Furthermore, having meals with loved ones and enjoying the social component of dining may improve the whole experience and develop a feeling of belonging and support.

Individuals undergoing gallbladder cancer therapy may improve their general health and well-being by having a good attitude toward food and nutrition.

CHAPTER NINE

Survival And Beyond

Life Following Cancer Treatment

Life following cancer treatment represents a huge adjustment for survivors. It is a period of adjustment, both physically and emotionally. Returning to normality may be difficult as survivors negotiate changes in their bodies, relationships, and daily routines. However, it is also a moment of optimism and rejuvenation, as survivors seize the chance to live their lives fully.

One of the most important components of life following cancer treatment is returning to regular follow-up consultations and tests. These consultations are critical for monitoring the survivor's health and finding any symptoms of cancer return early. During these follow-up appointments, healthcare practitioners may do physical exams, blood tests, imaging scans, and other testing to check that the survivor is still cancer-free. By being diligent with follow-up treatment, survivors may take proactive actions to preserve their health and well-being.

The Need For Regular Follow-Up Appointments And Screenings

Cancer survivors' long-term health depends on regular follow-up checkups and testing. These consultations let healthcare experts check for indicators of cancer recurrence or treatment problems. Early identification of cancer recurrence may dramatically improve results by allowing for timely intervention and therapy. Regular screenings may also help identify other health risks that may occur as a consequence of cancer therapy, such as heart disease or osteoporosis.

For many survivors, the prospect of cancer recurrence is daunting. However, maintaining consistency with follow-up treatment may bring peace of mind by ensuring that they are taking proactive actions to protect their health. Survivors must talk honestly with their healthcare provider about any concerns or symptoms they may have between consultations. Working together, survivors and their healthcare practitioners may create a personalized follow-up plan that addresses their specific needs and concerns.

Long-Term Dietary Concerns For Cancer Survivors

Cancer survivors' long-term health and well-being are heavily influenced by their diets. After treatment, survivors may confront new dietary concerns, including managing side effects, maintaining a healthy weight, and lowering the chance of cancer recurrence. Making educated food choices may help survivors improve their health and lower their chance of developing other chronic conditions.

One important aspect for cancer survivors is controlling treatment-related side effects that may impair their ability to eat effectively. For example, certain cancer therapies might produce nausea, taste changes, or trouble swallowing, making it difficult to maintain a healthy diet. In certain circumstances, survivors may benefit from consulting with a certified dietician, who may provide personalized dietary advice and support.

Emotional And Psychological Aspects Of Survivorship

The emotional and psychological components of surviving are as significant as the physical ones. Survivors may feel a variety of emotions as they navigate life following cancer treatment, including fear, worry, grief, anger, and uncertainty.

It is critical for survivors to recognize that their sentiments are normal and to seek help when necessary.

Many survivors find it beneficial to connect with other survivors who have had similar situations. Support groups, both in person and online, may foster a feeling of belonging and understanding. Individual counseling or therapy may also provide survivors with a secure environment in which to process their feelings and build coping techniques for stress and anxiety.

Resources And Support For Cancer Survivors

Cancer survivors may access a variety of tools and support services to assist them navigate life after treatment. These may include survivorship programs sponsored by hospitals or cancer centers that provide survivors with information, support, and resources targeted to their specific needs. Furthermore, national and local organizations such as the American Cancer Society and the Cancer Support Community provide a wide range of programs and services, such as support groups, educational seminars, and internet resources.

Survivors should also tap into their support networks, which include family, friends, and healthcare practitioners. Creating a strong support network may provide emotional support, practical aid, and companionship throughout the survival process. By using these tools and support services, survivors may improve their quality of life and flourish in the years after therapy.

CHAPTER TEN

Campaigning For Awareness And Prevention

Importance Of Increasing Awareness About Gallbladder Cancer

Raising awareness of gallbladder cancer is critical given its low prevalence but high fatality rate. Many patients are unaware of this kind of cancer until it is advanced, making treatment challenging. Individuals may improve their chances of effective treatment and survival by being more aware of potential signs and seeking medical help as soon as possible.

Awareness campaigns may also assist in clarifying myths and misunderstandings about gallbladder cancer. For example, many individuals may be unaware that certain risk factors, like as obesity, a high-fat diet, and gallstone production, might increase their chances of having this kind of cancer. Individuals may minimize their chance of having gallbladder cancer by being more aware of these risk factors.

Furthermore, increasing awareness may highlight the need for frequent health screenings and check-ups. Early detection of gallbladder cancer leads to much better treatment results. Encouraging people to have regular tests may lead to early identification and action, potentially saving lives.

Raising awareness of gallbladder cancer may also help patients and families form support networks. Dealing with a cancer diagnosis may be emotionally and mentally difficult, but knowing that others understand their situation can bring much-needed comfort and motivation.

By raising awareness of gallbladder cancer, we may eventually enhance early diagnosis, treatment results, and support networks for individuals afflicted by the illness.

Strategies For Encouraging Cancer Prevention In Communities

Preventing gallbladder cancer requires adopting initiatives that target modifiable risk factors and encourage healthy behaviors in communities. One such technique is to encourage people to maintain a healthy weight by engaging in regular exercise and eating a balanced diet. Obesity is a substantial risk factor for gallbladder cancer, therefore encouraging weight control may help minimize the disease's occurrence.

Another essential preventative approach is to educate people about the relationship between nutrition and gallbladder function. A diet strong in saturated fats and cholesterol increases the chance of developing gallstones, which are a precursor to gallbladder cancer. Encouraging individuals to eat fruits, vegetables, nutritious grains, and lean meats may help avoid gallstones and lower their risk of gallbladder cancer.

Furthermore, encouraging smoking cessation programs may help lower the incidence of gallbladder cancer since smoking is a proven risk factor for a variety of malignancies, including gallbladder cancer. Implementing tobacco control programs and giving support for quitting smoking may help communities avoid cancer.

Furthermore, improving access to healthcare services may aid in early identification and management for those at risk of developing gallbladder cancer. This involves making screening programs more inexpensive and accessible, as well as training healthcare practitioners to recognize and treat the signs and symptoms of gallbladder cancer.

By applying these techniques, communities may collaborate to lower the prevalence of gallbladder cancer and enhance overall public health outcomes.

Advocacy For Improved Access To Healthcare Services

Advocating for increased access to healthcare services is critical to ensure that all patients, regardless of socioeconomic position or geographic location, get prompt and high-quality treatment for gallbladder cancer. This involves campaigning for legislation that increases healthcare coverage while lowering obstacles to care, such as cost, transportation, and language challenges.

One method to advocate for improved healthcare access is to support efforts that enhance money for cancer research and treatment programs. By directing money to these areas, authorities may increase gallbladder cancer patients' access to cutting-edge therapies and interventions.

Furthermore, pushing for policies that promote healthcare workforce development may assist solve healthcare provider shortages in marginalized communities. This involves measures to educate and retain healthcare personnel, as well as incentives for practicing in regions with limited access to treatment.

Furthermore, lobbying for the use of telemedicine and telehealth services may enhance access to specialized treatment for those living in distant or rural locations. These technologies allow people to consult with healthcare experts remotely, minimizing the need for travel and increasing access to timely treatment.

Participating in advocacy initiatives at the local, state, and national levels may assist raise awareness about the significance of equal access to healthcare services for people with gallbladder cancer. Working together to lobby for policy reforms and resource allocation will guarantee that everyone has access to the treatment they need to prevent, diagnose, and treat gallbladder cancer.

Supporting Research And Innovation In Cancer Treatment

Supporting cancer research and innovation is crucial for improving patient outcomes in gallbladder cancer. Research is critical in discovering novel therapy options, understanding the underlying processes of cancer development, and creating tailored medicines to enhance patient outcomes.

One method to encourage research and innovation is to lobby for more funding for cancer research programs and institutes. Cancer research is funded by government agencies, private foundations, and pharmaceutical firms, and pushing for more expenditure in these areas may assist in speeding discovery and innovation.

Furthermore, sponsoring efforts that encourage cooperation between academics, physicians, and industry partners may aid in the translation of fundamental scientific findings into therapeutic applications. By encouraging multidisciplinary cooperation and information exchange, we can speed up the discovery of innovative gallbladder cancer therapies and interventions.

Furthermore, pushing for policies that shorten the regulatory approval process for cancer medications and therapies may help patients get innovative treatments faster. This involves campaigning for policies that prioritize patient outcomes and include patient feedback in the medication development process.

Engaging patients and their families in research may also assist in ensuring that research goals are in line with patients' needs and preferences. By integrating patients as research collaborators, we may create better patient-centered approaches to cancer therapy and care.

By funding cancer research and innovation, we may improve outcomes for people with gallbladder cancer and eventually strive toward a future in which this illness is more efficiently avoided, identified, and treated.

Empowering People To Take Control Of Their Health

Empowering people to take control of their health is critical for avoiding gallbladder cancer and improving patient outcomes. This entails equipping people with the information, skills, and tools they need to make informed choices about their health and wellness.

One strategy to empower people is to teach them about the risk factors for gallbladder cancer and how to lower their risk. This involves encouraging good lifestyle habits such as keeping a healthy weight, eating a balanced diet, exercising frequently, and abstaining from tobacco use.

Furthermore, providing patients with access to preventative healthcare services such as frequent screenings and check-ups may aid in the early detection of gallbladder cancer, while it is still curable. By encouraging people to prioritize their health and seek preventative care, we can increase early identification and treatment of gallbladder cancer.

Furthermore, educating people to advocate for themselves in the healthcare system may help them get prompt and appropriate treatment for gallbladder cancer. This involves training people how to successfully interact with healthcare practitioners, ask questions, and seek second views as needed.

Supporting patient empowerment entails tackling social and economic obstacles to healthcare access, such as poverty, prejudice, and a lack of health insurance. By fighting for policies that promote health equity and social justice, we can make the healthcare system more inclusive and accessible to everyone.

CONCLUSION

Dietary choices have an important influence on the development and treatment of gallbladder cancer. While the specific processes are not entirely known, research shows that some dietary components may increase the chance of getting gallbladder cancer, while others may protect against it.

A high diet of refined sugars, bad fats, and processed foods, along with a poor consumption of fruits, vegetables, and whole grains, has been linked to an increased risk of gallbladder cancer. Obesity and metabolic problems such as diabetes make this risk much higher.

In contrast, a diet high in fruits, vegetables, whole grains, and healthy fats like those found in fish and nuts may reduce the chance of getting gallbladder cancer. Furthermore, keeping a healthy weight via a balanced diet and regular exercise is critical for lowering the risk of obesity-related malignancies, such as gallbladder cancer.

While dietary changes alone may not prevent gallbladder cancer, they may improve general health and well-being, possibly lowering the chance of this fatal illness. Future research should concentrate on understanding the underlying processes that connect food to gallbladder cancer and creating tailored dietary therapies to reduce this risk.

THE END